Shibari

Japanese Bondage Techniques: Learn the Most Popular Japanese Art of Seduction

Contents

Book Description

You have probably come across people suspended in museums, clubs or stadiums and become fascinated, take the example of the Japanese models and how they play with ropes suspended in midair, apart from that you probably have witnessed a Shibari concert session and gained a hunger to know more of what it entails, well, you are in the right place! This book contains answers and puzzles that you may have about Japanese bondage techniques and how they have become a new world fantasy.

Shibari is the best recommendation a sex therapist will give you if you desire more pleasure and fun during intercourse, it is one of the best techniques that will spice up your sex life and also relax your body, many have given it a chance and never regret it, by reading the book you will be opening a new horizon of things you didn't even imagine of, the ropes, the knots, and the designs will keep you aroused and open to learning more on various techniques.

Shibari is not just like the rest of the seduction methods that you probably heard of or come across, it combines meditation, massage and seduction. By practicing the technique, you will be freeing your mind and body and generating a relaxation effect in you, the techniques laid out in this book will guide you on how to begin and what's needed, follow the preceding chapters and get to know more.

Shibari is a modern seduction technique that is meant to please both parties involved, in my journey as a Shibari student, I learnt all about the Japanese culture in relation to the technique and also gained vast familiarity and expertise since I learnt from the hands of the masters, my curiosity in Shibari has led me to new discoveries and innovations, I have analyzed and researched also from various sources globally and compiled my findings in this book.

Here are the topics covered:

Introduction to Shibari
Benefits of Shibari
Shibari patterns
Shibari techniques
The rigger (Nawashi)
Types of ropes used in Shibari

Chapter 1: Introduction to Shibari

Shibari the erotic art of seduction

Shibari is a form engaging art that involves submitting a subject to bondage by tying them up with ropes, also referred to as kinbaku by the Japanese culture. It involves three characters just like in painting that is the nawashi or rigger whom is the artist, the model that is the subject and the ropes which act as the paint in the art, besides that Shibari is an attractive art that sexually arouses its audience. It generally was adapted from the Hojo jutsu method derived from the Japanese; the Japanese used Hojo jutsu to respectfully withhold their captives by keeping them comfortable while at the same time holding them captive.

Compared to modern bondage methods such as hand cuffs or for example being tied down to a chair all day long, the Japanese would lay the captive on a bed and tie their hands to the head of the bed with one leg tied to the end instead of two. They would also build submission cages whereby; they would strip their captives naked and hang them suspending in midair.

The hojo jutsu technique survived to the late 1800s, after which Shibari was founded in the 1900s, Shibari being originally founded as an art, has since evolved into both a health benefit technique, sport and erotic tool, over the preceding chapters we shall be analysing and learning more on how Shibari is a health benefit, erotica and tool.

The rigger
The rigger also known as the nawashi is the artist behind tying kup the models, one is deemed to be a satisfied rigger after spending extensive years in study of the human body and how to tie different Japanese knots.

The ropes

The ropes to be used in Shibari have to be strong enough, they can be natural fiber with a diameter ranging from 7mm- 8mm, the standard feet of rope used during Shibari is 30 feet while the maximum is 69feet, the longer and stronger the rope, the better. Initially the form of rope used in Shibari is the jute rope.

8 benefits of Shibari for your health
Yes, just like the title says, Shibari for health benefits, You probably might be in curiosity as to how Shibari can save your life besides being an erotic art, or how exactly it can help improve your health, well In this chapter research records of the health benefits and side effects as experienced by the subject and nawashi have been compiled from sources all over the globe and extracted to the following ten points.

Shibari is a form of massage.
It is similar to the shiatsu massage In that it applies tension to the main pressure points of the body; the only difference is, the shiatsu method involves touching, rubbing and padding of the pressure points while Shibari involves applying tension to the pressure points by gliding a rope over them for some time. The pressure points include; shoulders, hips, ankles, the lower back and wrists.

Shibari helps reduce anxiety in the body.
According to the latest research on Shibari done by university of Wessex practitioners, a group of five women suffering from deep anxiety of the future volunteered as Shibari models in one of the town's museums, they had professional riggers train them as they entangled the ropes between them and stayed on the air for a maximum of one hour, moving and playing with the ropes each time they got tired, after the exercise they seemed to be livelier and optimistic, their minds and bodies were manipulated to relax as they wrestled with the ropes avoiding heavy tension on one area.

Improves circulation of the blood and other nutrients.

By submitting as a model in Shibari, your body will be freed from clogging, the blood transport utilities such as veins that transport blood and other nutrients such as food and gases throughout the whole body will be unclogged by the gliding of the ropes throughout the body, this will in turn help your body to be relieved of common illnesses such as arthritis and high blood pressure.

Liberates the body from stiffness on the neck and shoulders or back
By submitting the body to enormous pressure from the ropes or the strong sheets and the twisting involved the body muscles are bound to loosen up and become flexible, Shibari will also help in healing the sciatica disease whose symptoms are stiffness of one body part such as the legs followed by a sharp pain running over.

Helps in joining together of dislocated joints
As a form of massage, Shibari will also help in reaching deep beneath the skin and muscles then rubbing the dislocated joints together hence accelerating the healing, the ropes or tough sheets are able to dig deep in the body's flesh and gently squeeze over the bones.

Shapes your body with ease
With the constant twisting, stretching and bending your body is bound to burn a lot of calories and fats, practicing Shibari will leave your body in perfect form, you will save a lot of time and sweat from working out activities.

Improves the strength of your senses and spirituality
Shibari is a sexual arousal technique and massage, by practicing this art of rope bondage; you will be meditating and improving on your natural abilities to touch feel and predict. This can be well demonstrated by the professional Shibari models as their senses are always on top form; they climb hundreds of feet up a rope or tough plain sheet then play with the ropes courageously and precisely with no fear of falling off.

Helps in gaining a higher self esteem

By relaxing your body and mind, you are able to concentrate more on what you love doing, besides the concentration on what you do best you are also able to accept who you are by meditation.

Common forms of Shibari patterns

One wrist tying method also known as Kakate Kubi form of Shibari
This happens when the rigger ties up one hand skillfully with fine knots to either the shoulder or any other body part; the wrist is bound in such a way that the rest of the arm is free from ropes. It is also important to note that while tying, pass the rope behind the joint.

Both wrists tied method also known as Ryoute kubi form of Shibari
Tying both wrists is also similar to tying one wrist, the rope is passed behind the joint and tied in such a way that it will not cause any injury or harm to the model.

Both hands behind the back binding method also known as gote form of Shibari

This is the trickiest binding in Shibari, a lot of riggers make mistakes that later lead to consequences such as nerve compression and poor circulation all over the body. The rope should avoid nerves and joints always. In this method the model knots should be strong enough that they can suspend the models entire body without causing any harm.

Diamond tying/ turtle binding method also known as hishi nawa form of Shibari
In this form of binding, the rigger tries his best to shame the model with knots and strips running over their sexual organs.

Apart from that there are other patterns ranging to over ten thousand, Most of the patterns require flexible models and take time to complete. However, in this book we shall be looking into the basic techniques that lead to the expertise techniques.

Chapter 2: Gote Shibari (the boxed tie)

Gote Shibari
In this technique the model folds their hands on their back creating a square between their shoulders and elbows; the rigger then ties them up in such a way that the model looks as if there wearing a vest but their chest is not crossed with the ropes, this method is for displaying the front chest of the model in such a way that the audience has a full view of the front.

Characters/ items involved:
Rigger
Model (female)
ropes
Blind fold

Other requirements
The model should be either dressed in tight light clothing, no clothes or a bikini only. This is to enhance the art to be more appealing and exotic.
The rigger should wear a short sleeved t-shirt or shirt that will not cause interruptions while tying the knots.

Procedure:

Have the model sit on a carpet facing away from you in an open space where stretching won't be a glitch then tie the blind fold to the model.

Move the models hands to their back that they may overlie against each other (as if hands fold from the back) forming a square between the shoulders and hands. The model should have her left hand on her right elbow and the right hand on left elbow.

Join the two ends of the rope together that it may be comprise of two to make the tying more effective and stronger.

Tie the double rope on the hands avoiding the joints; that is in the middle of the elbows and wrists. Don't make it too tight though, you don't want to hurt your model.

After binding the hands to the back forming a square, don't cut the double rope yet, run it slightly below the left shoulder to avoid contact with the joint moving across the lower chest so it crosses slightly below the right shoulder joint then bring the rope through the extension to the left shoulder, don't make it too tight, follow the track back from the right shoulder to the left then through the knot made over the right extension. That will be your second knot, run the rope over the knot to make it firmer, you can do this even twice.

The next step should be to make sure that the ropes are lying flat not over each other, do this by moving your fingers through the extensions passing through the chests and the shoulders, while doing that, hold the models shoulders that they may be comfortable and not facing the wrong way.

After that take the rope and pass it under the right arm, make sure the rope is still in double form and passes alternatively over the bicep then lie the model on your chest that you may have a view of the chest, pull the rope gently you just drove under the arm over the junction of the chest and arm and pull it from under the extensions across the chest, don't tighten the rope, let it lie over the extension.

After that hopefully your rope will not be over like mine, in case it's over no need to panic, grab another piece of rope. Just like in the first case hold the two ends of your rope together to form one double rope and make a loop, on the rope that ended on the models body, make a knot at each of the overlying rope and submerge them in your new rope loop, the loop should be firm enough.

After joining the two ropes together in a tight loop, drive the rope through (under the arm) and pull it back to the hands. And that's it, make sure that the knots are not underneath as they will harm the model.

The technique is good especially if the model is to be suspended; it will take some time to have the ropes unsealed from the model's body.

Chapter 3: Shibari Futomomo

Shibari futomomo (leg bondage)

Also called Shibari futomomo is one of the best Shibari techniques that will make your spouse speak in tongues is the leg bondage technique, this is whereby the model's legs are tied apart to either their thighs then to their back or on a chair or suitable frame, the model is then left with legs wide open arousing their audience. Combining the futomomo and the Shibari chest tying methods the result is usually a masterpiece.

Requirements
Rope approximately 30 feet long
Blind folds if you want to make the act juicier

Other requirements
The model can choose from no clothing to light clothing or just a bikini.
The rigger has to be dressed in a way that they will have no interruptions while tying the model.

Procedure
The model and the rigger work while lying down to make extra room for movement, using the rope the rigger finds the mid by placing both ends of the rope together then takes the curved mind to work with it as a double stripped rope.

The rigger then makes a collar tie (this is when the tails of the rope are passed through the centre piece curve) above the models ankle after which the model presses her ankle close to her hip, the rigger then makes the first wrap from where the hip and the thigh meet right in the groove note that the wraps are double striped.

The rigger then proceeds on tying the wraps evenly spaced round the leg and thigh avoiding the rope from overlying on top of each other till he or she almost reaches the knee joint, remember in Shibari always avoid tying up on the joints, it might eventually lead to injuries or severe consequences, also remember to tighten the wraps. An averagely tall person should have four to five wraps.

The rigger then makes a manta (making a loop by passing the rope over the extension of the first string and then driving it under so that the first extension wrap lies on it) then over again so the first strip extension is held firmly by the rope, the rope which should be now facing downward the tails of the rope are then moved underneath the band, the tails are then moved across the diagonal strip coming down from the first wrap then passed over and underneath the second strip, you will notice that the perpendicular strip is now held at the centre of the two loops and now the rope tails are facing downwards.

The rigger then makes similar approaches to the next wraps before the last wrap, for easy understanding this means that the rigger makes mantas until he or she reaches the final wrap. On the final wrap encircle the rope to the strip then bring it underneath so it pops on the other side.

After the rope pops out of the other end, the rigger builds mantas upwards going centreline remember that when making mantas ensure that you loop the diagonal strips by looping them around on both sides, this involves moving the ropes to the next strip, encircling the strip then going across the centreline and encircling the strips again, also ensure that no rope is overlying on top of the other or hanging loose.

After finishing the last loop, the rigger must now lock the loop, the loop is tied on the final strip and the remaining piece of rope is used to make mantas down the wraps again.

This is a great method of dominance during intercourse, the female's bottom is exposed perfectly and also allows the tying of the legs to a chair or suspension ring, this exposes a better view of the ladies centre region as intended.

Chapter 4: Shibari koshinawa

Shibari koshinawa (hip harnessing)
In this technique, concentration lies on the central region, that is the hips, the rigger ensures that the curves are well pressed out and cause an arousal effect on the audience, the hips are tied together in a way that only the hips move and later suspended.

Requirements
30 feet rope
Spacious floor
Rigger/ nawashi
model
Other requirements
an additional rope if need be
suspension ring if the model wishes to be suspended
Procedure
The first step the rigger takes is to perform a single collar standard tie on the hips placing the rope (double stripped) between the two hip bones and running the most of the prominent parts of the butt. It is very important that the integrity of and safety of this tie interlocks the bite by passing the rope through, firm tension is required to maintain effectiveness.

The rigger then precedes by making two parallel wraps around the thighs below the models private region diagonally to the strip on the hipbone that now there may be for strips that are not lying against each other but are touching. The rigger then moves the rope around the leg again creating four lines of ropes round one leg.

The rigger then closes the three wraps on one leg, that is; the top strip that is tied on the hip bone and the other two strips tied on the thigh and touching the first strip, he or she does this by running their fingers underneath the parallel strips then pulling the rope from below then going over them again and pulling the rope again from underneath, this forms a loop by which this strips underlie, the rigger then keeps running his fingers underneath the ropes to ensure there is no point where they overlie against each other, also remember that the knots should not lie underneath to avoid injury.

After looping the two parallel strips the rigger then moves upwards and drives the rope beneath the first strip then pulls the rope which makes the loop carrying the two parallel strips go upwards. The rigger then finishes on the first leg by performing a friction (manta knots) then goes to the other leg and performs a similar way to the first leg.

After finishing the second leg, the rigger moves the rope round again the butt of the model and then makes another knot to the center, this forms a bigger knot than two of the knots on the junction of each hipbone and thigh, the rigger then precedes by running the rope over the left hip of the model over the back and over again the right hip then back to the center knot, the rope should lie on the hips as a tie lies to the collar bone.

The rigger then makes another manta on the center knot and this time drives the rope over the right hip bone across the back over the left hipbone and back to the centre knot, the rigger make another manta and then wraps the remaining rope round the suspension after which he or she locks the knot tightly, make sure that the knots don't lie underneath and that the strings don't overlie on top of each other. The rigger has now finished their work.

Suspension know can be made at the center, the knots will withhold the entire mass of the body, many creative riggers have mixed up different Shibari techniques such as this with the breast tying style and come up with some awesome stuff. This technique holds the butt's curves tightly and makes it possible to tie the hips on a suspension.

Chapter 5: Teppou Shibari

Teppou Shibari
Teppou is the Japanese way of saying a gun; the technique involves tying the hands to the back so that they resemble the shape of a gun. In this type of bondage one hand is tied over the shoulder of the model while the other hand is tied folded up and under the back. The main aim of this technique is to have the models chest open with no ropes to the front unlike the gote Shibari technique.

Requirements
2 Ropes 30 feet
Rigger
Model
The scene requires the rigger to be comfortably dressed and in a spacious room.
Procedure

As the rigger, have the model sited on the floor with you while she faces away, this gives you a clear view of her back.

The rigger starts by making a single collar loop by the wrist and locks the double strip roped formed as a result of the curve on the mid of the rope, the next thing is to take the models hand over her shoulder that she may have her hand touching her back, as you do this, please don't strain your model as flexibility varies in different people, straining or forcing may lead to dislocations or other severe consequences.

The rigger then holds the wrist in a way that it is in contact with the shoulder then runs the rope over binding them together, wrap the wrist and arm again this time crossing the first extension, after crossing again pass the rope over and underneath the two extensions making a manta.

The rigger then brings the second hand backwards, be careful so you don't spoil the shape of your model and glides the rope on the middle of the wrist and elbow avoiding the joints then passing it under the arm over the bicep then back to the middle of the elbow and wrist, the rigger then runs the rope over the bicep and under the arm the looping it over the suspension rope from the other hand, notice that all ties have four strips now.

The rigger will has now run out of rope or is almost if they did it right with a 30feet rope, he or she joins the rope to another to increase the length then moves to the other hand which is the upper one then wraps the rope under underneath the bicep and over the elbow slightly above to increase the firmness of the joint after that looping them together then back to the lower hand and glide the rope over the bicep, underneath the arm twice, the rigger then loops the joint tightly avoiding injury to the model after which he follows up the suspension rope making periodic mantas till the rope is finished.

This method will release tension from the front chest of the model and also mark as a sign of submission to their sexual partner, the model can have her back tied to the wall or suspension string to make it more fun.

Chapter 6: Ganraptor Shibari

Ganraptor Shibari
In this technique the rigger ties the models legs in anticipation of suspension. The rope strips must be tight enough and firm so as to handle the total weight when suspended. After finishing this technique, a rope is then tied to the knot on the hip so that the model can be suspended by her legs and hips.
Requirements
30feet rope
The rigger
The model
The suspension mechanism can also be done outside under a tree.
Procedure
The rigger first runs the first rope over the hips of the model making a four strip colour then using the second rope, runs it over the big toe of the model to until the ends of the rope meet, the big toe should now be lying in the middle of the two strips.

The rigger then takes the two tails of the rope to form one double sided rope and wraps them underneath the ankle then over to meet the first extension of the rope from the big toe. Remember that the rope should not be in contact with the ropes to avoid the joint.

The rigger then passes the rope underneath the foot then over the foot again this time heading underneath the ankle to make a second strip, He or she then moves the rope over the foot again this time passing it underneath the first strip then underneath then comes up and ties the rope to the second strip across the ankle, it is important that in this point the rigger checks if there is any rope lying against another, if so it must be amended to be straight.

After passing the rope underneath the first double strip running across the ankle the rigger then pulls the rope and runs it over the second double strip across the ankle and makes the third double strip over the ankle and passes it underneath the middle strip running over the top of the ankle.

The rigger now drives the rope over the foot and underneath, this time the rope doesn't go over but drives the rope underneath both the two strips and creates a loop, he or she later takes of the single strip of rope over the big toe and ties to the rope from the foot, the rigger makes sure that there are no overlying strips and no knots lying underneath, the foot binding is now complete.

If the model consents to suspension the earlier rope tied across the hips is tied to the branch of the tree then to the foot rope, the rigger then pulls the rope till it is now tied to the strip running across the hip bones.

Chapter 7: Takate Kote

Takate Kote (Tying of the female chest in Shibari)
In this technique the rigger binds the models breasts and hands in such a way that the model cannot make any movement and that the breasts are held firmly squeezed out and pointing out, as you remember we said in the first chapter that Shibari is meant to shame the captive but also in a way that they also enjoy the bondage. Most riggers and audience like this technique because it exposes the captive's chest to vulnerability from the audience.

Requirements
Ropes
Blind fold if need be
Procedure
Have the model dressed in tight clothing and the rigger in a comfortable sleeveless t-shirt or shirt.

Hold the ropes end together that they may form a curve at the middle just like in the gote Shibari method; hold the rope by the curve so as to make a double sided rope. In this method the model does not have to sit down but has to raise their hands to prevent constant interruption from the rigger.

While the model is facing backwards away from you who in this scenario is the rigger, move the rope by the middle under their breasts gently avoiding overlapping to their backs then pass the double rope inside the curve, pull it to make it tight but not model-unfriendly tight, run the double rope again from the loop to under the models breasts to her back where the first loop is then drag the rope through the second loop formed while making the second extension, make sure that the extensions have not over lied on each other.

Run the rope under the models left arm below the armpit that it may run over her breasts and under the right armpit to the loop centre on the models back through the extension to the left you just created, drive the rope again from the loop below the right armpit, over the models breast and under her left armpit heading back through the extension you just created heading to the right arm make sure you roll the rope over the extension, check again for any overlying extensions and fix by running your fingers over them again.

You should now have noticed that you have two loops lying on the back of the model, two extensions run to the left and two extensions to the right with all of them having four stripes of ropes.

Move your fingers through the extensions and pull the ends through the other two loops to make a big loop then tighten it by pulling the rope steadily till the loops are now in contact with each other.

After that you probably notice that your double rope is getting short that is if yours is 5ft like mine, now drive the rope over the left side of the neck to the lower extension of the breasts. If you have reached your ropes end then make two knots on the two ends of the rope, grab the other rope, hold it by its middle curve to make a double strip rope then loop the end of the finished ropes, this should help you in bringing in the new rope, make sure the knots are not underneath so that you don't harm the model.

After adjusting continue across the neck over the first extension to the bottom four strip extension, on the bottom extension pass the rope underneath it, move the rope up heading to the top strip and pass the rope underneath making sure that the extension from the neck you just made is now in between where you're passing the rope and one breast.

After pulling the rope from underneath, cross it over the extension from the neck to underneath the top strip then pull heading underneath the bottom strip, continue checking that no rope underlies over the other, pull the rope from underneath the second strip and move it to the curved loop on the cleavage, pass it under the rope curve then pull.

This is the tricky part, make sure all strips don't lie on top of each other or sideways from each other, drive the rope across the other side of the neck to the back, and bind the rope to the knot behind, check if there are any ropes underlying on top of each other. You can run the rope underneath and over the loop until you feel it's strong enough.

Drive the rope across one shoulder and let it pass underneath the top strip then to the back again pass the rope over the first two strips of the four strip extension then under the other two, head down the other four strip extension and pass over the first two and underneath the other two, cross the big loop to the bottom four strip extension and pass over the first two and underneath the other two to make it firmer do the same for the upper four strips following the pattern.

After, drive the rope over the shoulder to the top strip and run the rope underneath then pull it back over the shoulder to the back tie like you did in the other side, after you're done, tie both ends of the rope and that's it, the breasts should be perfectly squeezed out.

This technique exposes the female breasts fully; it also exerts more pressure on the firmness of the breasts, you can also combine it with the first method that involves tying both of the hands on the back in a comfortable way, by doing this the model will be submitting to total dominance of her chest.

Conclusion

Shibari is a modern new age form of erotic art massage which many in the world are still not familiar with, it involves bondage and submission to special ropes referred to as jute that origin from the Japanese, the artist binding the model is known as the rigger.

The Japanese adapted the erotica technique from kinbaku, which was a tactical way to bind and hold their captives during the 1800s. The Japanese would shamefully tie up their captives and suspend them in public areas where in some scenarios they would be whipped till they revealed what their real intentions were.

However, the Japanese soon realized that some of their captives were enjoying the torture, a Japanese man known as Seiu Ito, was fascinated by how the captives had evolved to liking the bondage, he started studying the technique and combining it with art till finally he came up with Shibari. Seiu is now a celebrated figure and referred to as the father of Shibari, his works have been compiled along walls, books and traditional Japanese articles.

Shibari has been proved to be good for health and also meditation; it involves subjecting the body to flexibility and tension which in turn relaxes the nerves and deep tissues, the technique is widely adapted in neuron therapy whereby the patients undergo tying of their body parts to help in assembling dislocated joints, apart from being used in the healing process, you will also note that night clubs especially in the U.K are adapting the style as a way of attracting attention.

As technology races with time, there are also new innovations that have been developed such as the Shibari sticks e,g the hentai magic stick that is attached to the clitoris of the woman.

This has led to the up rise of controversy since the machines are not able to perform as the ropes do. The Japanese association of Nawashi teachers has termed the gadgets as an abolishment to the Shibari nature.

As we move on to the next century, there are different new Shibari techniques being discovered, currently there are over ten thousand ways to bind a model in captivity but the most methods are for trained professionals only, However, it is still emphasized to practice Shibari naturally with a rigger to train you no matter how simple the technique might be, remember that people have different levels of flexibility also, what a person might do another might not be able to do.

Shibari is now a profession to many, just like it takes creativity to come up with a masterpiece, so does Shibari, nowadays there are Shibari concerts held all over the world, there are masters in the field who make some bucks tying up people, it can be a good hobby to master.

Despite the numerous positivity Shibari carries, it has been misunderstood as an evil act by many since they proclaim that the act incorporates tying and shame that go hand in hand with evil, but there is no justification in this, the model consents to being tied up and held captive, the model is the one who has most of the fun.

www.ingramcontent.com/pod-product-compliance
Lightning Source LLC
Chambersburg PA
CBHW061950280526
45787CB00004B/1796